Dirty Genes Solution

The Revolutionary Approach to Addressing the Root Cause of Illness and Enhancing Your Well-being

By

Mark R. Dickson

Disclaimer

Copyright © by Mark R. Dickson 2024.
All rights reserved.

Table of Contents

Disclaimer

Introduction

Chapter 1:

Your Genes are Not Your Destiny

Chapter 2:

What Axactly is a "Dirty Gene,"

Chapter 3:

Various Types of Genes, and What They Do

Chapter 4:

Techniques for Having Positive Impact On Your Genes for Better

Chapter 5:

Fit-Genes Customized Genetic Health and Wellbeing Assessment

Chapter 6:

How to Clean Your Genes with the Soak and Scrub Method

Chapter 7:

Heart Problems: What Exactly is Heart Disease (Cardiovascular)?

Chapter 8:

Symptoms and causes of heart problems

Chapter 9:

Role of Nutrition in Gene Optimization
    Practical Strategies for A Gene-Friendly Diet
    Meal Plans and Recipes

Introduction

In a world where our genes are often seen as the unchangeable scripts of our health story, "Dirty Genes: A Breakthrough Program to Treat the Root Cause of Illness and Optimize Your Health" invites you to reconsider this narrative. Imagine stepping into a bustling kitchen filled with diverse ingredients, each holding the potential to influence the symphony of your genes. Meet Emma, a vibrant individual navigating the labyrinth of health misinformation, who discovers the transformative power of nutrition on her genetic blueprint.

Emma, like many, once believed that her genetic fate was a predetermined path, resistant to the choices she made on her dinner plate. However, as she dove into the pages of this groundbreaking book, she unearthed the truth –

that our genes are not dictators but collaborators in a dynamic dance with the foods we choose to consume.

As Emma experimented with nutrient-rich meals, she witnessed a shift in her well-being, realizing that her daily choices acted as conductors orchestrating the expression of her genes. The journey unfolds through captivating narratives of real-life individuals, illuminating the diverse ways in which dirty genes can be cleansed, paving the way for a healthier and more vibrant life.

Join Emma and others on this exploration of the intricate relationship between nutrition and genes. "Dirty Genes" offers not just a book, but a roadmap to understanding the melody within, where the language of genes meets the artistry of a well-balanced plate. Embark on a transformative odyssey that challenges common misconceptions and empowers you to script your health narrative in collaboration with the symphony of your own unique genetic composition.

Chapter 1:

Your Genes are Not Your Destiny

Many of us have spent our entire lives believing that we have little say over the state of our own health. We feel that because of our DNA, we cannot modify our bodies or our health. It is easy to reject the role of our lifestyle, throw our hands up in the air, and claim that nutrition, exercise, and self-care are unimportant if we come from a family with similar health conditions. If we are overweight or diabetic, and we come from a family that struggles with these diseases. We believe that a specific outcome is predetermined for us, and our beliefs are confirmed.

The truth is that we have a substantial amount of control over our health. Our genetic makeup cannot be changed, but the way we eat, move and live can all have a big impact on our genes and the level of expression they can reach. Now, I'd want to talk on the aforementioned topic." To paraphrase a popular statement, "My genes are not my destiny." Repeat after me.

Continue reading to get more information about:

Nature versus nurture.
Epigenetics
SNPs, or single nucleotide polymorphisms, are activities that can alter your genes.

Let's get started!

Nature Versus Nurture

The debate has raged for millennia, but I believe we have finally found a solution: nurture. People in the same family may have the same health problems because they promote the same types of habits and ways of life.

It was a bit of an anticlimactic moment in both the history of medicine and the history of the planet when scientists finally mapped the human genome in 2003 and discovered that humans have between 20,000 and 25,000 genes, rather than the higher number that was previously predicted. The discovery of the genome resulted in very little change in the treatments utilized for health concerns and chronic diseases, despite the fact that some genetic variations are clearly responsible for specific diseases.

It has come to our attention that a person's genes do not hold all of the answers. They could load the weapon, but the environment is what ultimately pulls the trigger. Another way to think about this is to consider your DNA as a bookcase filled with books, with the environment determining which books are read.

It is currently estimated that your genes are responsible for about 10% of diseases, with environmental variables accounting for the other 90%. The good news is that you have a significant amount of control over your environment. That's so encouraging!

Epigenetics

The term "epigenetics" refers to an environmental element that influences gene expression. Its literal meaning is "on top of genetics," and the term originates from that statement. How does the body decide which genes should be expressed?

Which one should be silenced? In addition to methylation and other biochemical activities, our bodies contain several different mechanisms that can communicate with our DNA. These include changes to histones. This occurs continuously in each and every cell.

The study of epigenetics helps us better comprehend the dynamic link that occurs between our genes and the environment. The way we live has a big impact on our overall health. When you hear about research claiming that eating more vegetables or indulging in high-intensity interval training is good for your health, one of the reasons is that these lifestyle behaviors influence your genetic expression in favor of health and longevity. The disease may cause these genes to become dormant.

What's the deal with SNPs?

The study of SNPs, also known as single nucleotide polymorphisms, is the most recent development in genetics research and is widely studied in functional medicine. A single nucleotide polymorphism, or SNP (pronounced "snip"), is a variant in which one DNA base is exchanged with another. In the great scheme of things, single nucleotide polymorphisms (SNPs) are the methods by which humans adjust to changing environments and conditions across time. However, because the human environment has evolved considerably faster than our DNA, some of the SNPs meant to provide protection may actually cause difficulties. One way to think about this phenomenon is as a mismatch in the epigenetic coding.

Let us take a moment to discuss methylation. The addition of a methyl group to a molecule is performed using a simple biochemical technique known as methylation. The body does this to cleanse itself, generate neurotransmitters, appropriately metabolize amino acids, and regulate which genes are switched on and off.

You may be familiar with MTHFR, which stands for methylene tetrahydrofolate reductase. MTHFR is an important enzyme in the methylation process.. To function effectively, MTHFR requires folate, vitamin B12, and others minerals. SNPs can be discovered in a considerable proportion of the population's MTHFR genes (the code that instructs the body to produce this enzyme).

There is little proof that MTHFR SNPs influence methylation, but this is frequently only the case when environmental factors are also present, such as eating a poor diet low in B vitamins or being exposed to more pollutants than the body can process. An MTHFR SNP does not require a low-functioning methylation cycle. Why? Epigenetics.

I just wanted to take a moment to discuss the power that lies within our ideas. Our epigenetics are influenced by how we think about our bodies and health. If test results show that we have the

MTHFR SNP or the BRCA gene, both of which are linked to breast cancer, we may have concerns about our future health. This information is causing anxiety, which is affecting our health negatively.

Especially these days, when we have access to so much information about our genetic composition, it is critical that we appreciate the connection that exists between the mind, body, and spirit. In my line of employment, I operate on the edge of legality. I believe that genetic information can give us helpful insights and pieces of the puzzle that is your health, but I also want to treat you as a whole person, not just your genetics. There is no certainty that a person will acquire a disease simply because they carry a gene or a variant in a gene. We will have to extend our perspective.

Next Steps
When it comes to giving your genes the conditions they require to thrive, it all boils down to the core lifestyle choices you practice.

These are the practices I discuss with patients on a regular basis and write about on my website. I am talking about:

- The food that people consume.
- The water we consume and the air we breathe
- Our exposure to dangerous compounds and polluted air
- How much we exercise and how often we move also play a role.
- The duration and depth of our sleep, respectively (link to sleep article).
- Our stress levels and how well we can manage them through self-care.
- The current state of our microbiome (microbial community)

In addition, epigenetics influences how features are passed down through generations. Your offspring will inherit your epigenetic expression, which will affect the genes they inherit from you. If you take care of yourself now, you will be better able to provide for your children and grandchildren in the future. This third factor provides a tremendous incentive for many people to adopt additional health-promoting practices.

Chapter 2:

What Axactly is a "Dirty Gene,"

According to the definition, a dirty gene is one whose function is hampered either by mutations at birth or by attitude, dietary and lifestyle choices, and environmental contaminants.

One person feels that in order to improve one's health, one should make more efforts in the areas of lifestyle, nutrition, stress management, thinking, and the use of toxin-free alternatives. "When you're born with a lot of dirty SNP's, you need to make higher efforts toward health." "When you're born with a bunch of unclean SNPs, you need to take extra steps toward health," according to one researcher."Dirty Genes" are genes that don't function properly in our biochemical pathways. This is either because they lack a critical enzyme or cofactor required for peak performance, or because other environmental factors are interfering with their capacity to fulfill their intended function.

When the normal, healthy function of a gene that has not been altered is hampered by variables such as nutritional deficiencies, environmental contaminants, stress, or any combination of these factors, the gene is considered "dirty."

"A gene can be dirty from birth because of an SNP, or it can become dirty as a result of exposure to mold, pollutants, or infection." The dirt has an influence on the gene's ability to function normally.

"A dirty gene is one that has to be cleansed and scrubbed," as the saying goes.

And here is the definition of a dirty gene that I like best because it is simple and concise:

A "dirty gene" is a gene that is not functioning optimally.

What effect does gene contamination have?

It is incapable of operating.
Work is not done because it does not perform properly.

Minor symptoms start to appear.
Because a single gene cannot accomplish its role, other genes, whether one or twenty in number, are recruited to help.
These genes are overused and eventually tired.
They begin to show soiling symptoms.
When you hear language like "more and more random symptoms are occurring," think about a chronic illness.
As some genes lose vigor, others emerge to take their place. These other genes are upset about it and express their unhappiness by generating noise.
When significant symptoms arise, seek emergency care.

It is preferable to find the dirt early on and remove it, right?

How can you do it if you don't know what the dirt is?
How do you accomplish that if you don't know which symptoms are linked to specific genes?

How are you expected to accomplish this if you don't know what these genes do, how they want to function, or how they become contaminated?
A gene (and the enzyme it produces) does not operate optimally if either of the following is true:

lacking vitamins and minerals to help activate the enzyme that it produces contains a variant or SNP that affects its shape, which then affects its ability to perform a function blocked by something - such as heavy metals, infections, chemicals, or other hormones lacks enough material to build with - such as lacking protein (methionine, tyrosine, tryptophan) has too much

material that inundates it - such as folic acid,
methionine a lack of material.

Chapter 3:

Various Types of Genes, and What They Do

Before we go into the many types of genetic material, let's first learn a little more about how genes work. When we learn that something--whether it's a trait like having blue eyes or a diagnosis like heart disease--is genetic, we frequently imagine our parents or grandparents handing it down like an undesirable inheritance. This could be a physical characteristic, such as blue eyes, or a medical condition, such as heart trouble.

On the other hand, there is usually more going on at the molecular level than is realized. Deoxyribonucleic acid, also known as DNA, is a chemical found in all of our cells, particularly in histones. It is transcribed by your cytoplasm and contains a code and instructions that provide each of us with our unique identities while distinguishing humans, animals, and plants.

Although no two people, including identical twins, have the same DNA or RNA sequence, all DNA is composed of the same four building blocks: adenine, cytosine, guanine, and thymine. Base pairs are formed when each chromosome combines with other chromosomes given by the reproductive partner.

In other words, the female supplies one chromosome while the father contributes the other to the offspring. This unique set of chromosomes forms a gene, and each gene has its own set of introns, exons, and a variety of other essential components.

Certain chromosomes appear to be more important than others, whereas others tend to melt together. This is due to the fact that there are numerous types of single genes, each of which deals with the interaction of two chromosomes and is manifested as a phenotype in a unique manner.

A phenotype is a specified trait that may be ascertained by observation. Phenotypes can occur in both plants and animals. The color of one's Phenotypes include things like one's hair, height, and the amount of clotting factor in their blood.

Gene Flow Biosciences, a biotechnology company, is doing research into the possibility of producing a medicine that targets the genes responsible for aging in humans. Because there are so many different gene types and genetic variations, let's start with a detailed explanation of the five most essential gene groups.

1. Genes that complement one another

Complementary genes require the cooperation of two dominant genes to produce a specific phenotype. In other words, both genes must be present at the same time for the desired phenotype to develop; otherwise, it will not be created. A single gene, or a combination of one dominant and one recessive gene, is insufficient to complete the task. Both dominant genes are helpful to each other.

2. Genes Considered Extra

Complementary genes are those that work together to produce a specific trait. Supplemental genes differ significantly from complementary genes. Supplemental genes are made up of two genes: one is a dominant gene that can express itself independently, and the other is a gene with the capacity to express itself. However, in order to function, it must be combined with an existing gene. In this case, the combination of the two genes may cause the development of a completely new trait or phenotype.

Mating two mice, one black and the other albino is a common example of this gene type. The albino mouse cannot produce a colored coat on its own; but, when bred with the black mouse, the offspring's coat color is neither black nor white, but rather a new hue that is somewhere in the middle: brown.

3. Duplicate genes.

The presence of duplicate genes is compatible with their name. It occurs when two dominant and recessive genes exhibit themselves simultaneously. One does not need the other to display a given phenotype since each has individually picked how they wish to express themselves and will do so regardless of the other. As a result, one does not require the other to have a specific phenotype.

The ability of these genes to reproduce phenotypic features is an intriguing thought.
Dr. Francis Collins' article explains the downsides of possessing duplicate clotting factors or insulin-producing genes, which might result in serious health problems. In light of this, the question arises: why has evolution not eliminated potentially hazardous duplicate genes from the gene pool by now?

4. Genes Made of Polymers

Polymeric genes, also known as additive genes, are similar to duplicate genes in that they have an additive or compounding effect on one another. However, polymeric genes do not necessarily include a pair of genes that express themselves in the same way.

Another example is summer squash, which is slightly more technical in nature. An essay published on biologydiscussion.com discusses how the combination of two separate squash shapes—spherical and cylindrical—created an entirely new squash shape known as discoid.

5. Sex-Linked Genes

These genes affect the human body's X or Y chromosomes, which are known as the sex chromosomes, and are responsible for defining sex as well as how distinct traits are inherited based on sex. Even recessive features found on X chromosomes in XX individuals (females) are more likely to be absent in XY individuals, who only have one X chromosome.

Color blindness is a well-known example of this phenomenon. Despite the fact that the genes that cause color blindness are recessive, a colorblind mother (XX) and a non-colorblind father (XY) can have a colorblind son. This is due to the son having only one copy of the X chromosome. As a result, it is likely that recessive genes will continue to be expressed.

Mutations

Genes can change structure over time, and only a tiny number of genes differ between individuals. This is because some genes are susceptible to mutations, which alter the structures generated by other genes. As an example, the SIRT6 gene is a gene that plays an important role in the regulation of our aging process by repairing DNA damage that accumulates over the course of our lives. The study by Genflow Biosciences discovered that centenarians have mutations in this gene. These tiny modifications to the SIRT6 gene improve its ability to repair DNA, slowing the aging process.

Genflow Bioscience believes that aging is not a natural process and that it can be slowed or prevented completely by giving gene therapy in the form of more copies of the centenarian variation of the SIRT6 gene. As generations pass, many sorts of mutations occur, causing the gene pool to gradually shift over time.

Although gene mutations have been linked to diabetes, cancers, breast cancer, other cancer cells, and sickle cell anemia, all of which impair hemoglobin synthesis, chromosomal translocation, and environmental factors also play a part in their development.

Chapter 4:

Techniques for Having Positive Impact On Your Genes for Better

Like the rest of us, perhaps, you have resolved to have a happy and healthy life in 2019. Though the grocery store's salad section is definitely disorganized and your gym may be a bit busier, everything is done with good intentions. But in light of the present health-consciousness, it's important to keep in mind that leading a healthy lifestyle is about more than just your scale numbers.

Our genes can benefit from changes in our behavior and way of life!
A healthy diet, regular exercise, getting enough sleep, avoiding stress, and discovering joy throughout the day are all underlying factors that contribute to our general well-being.

Remarkably, current studies suggest that positive adjustments in behavior and lifestyle may also have a genetic component. Given that every one of us is born with a fixed genome, this may seem contradictory, but the degree of activity in our genes can change.

The study of possible modifications to gene expression that may not need alterations to the underlying DNA sequence, or a phenotypic shift without a genotype shift, that alters how cells interpret their genes is known as epigenetics.
Modern research focuses on the epigene, a complex protein sheath that envelops DNA and regulates the expression of several genes. This genetic activity is dynamic and ever-changing, reacting to the data we provide our bodies. Although identical twins have the same genome at birth, by the time they are in their senior year of life, their genes have responded to their experiences, leaving their genetic readouts no more similar than those of two siblings who are not twins.

How then may one enhance their genetic makeup?

These six techniques will ensure that your way of life is positively influencing your genetic makeup.

1. See every day as an ongoing feedback loop. Aim for a higher ratio of positive to negative feedback.

2. Don't restrict your 'positive input' to kale consumption. It could be anything from eating wholesome foods to developing a positive outlook to dressing in something that makes you feel amazing. Having fun during the day is just as important as finishing your tasks.

3. Make a small adjustment. To keep your day exciting, give yourself time for socializing, alone time, and recreational activities.

4. Be mindful of your physical form. Eat only when you are hungry and don't stay up until your body naturally feels tired—no, this doesn't mean you should always take a sleep when you're tired—you get the idea. Your boss would probably not approve.

5. Lessen your anxiety. Stress reduction manifests itself immediately at the cellular level. If you find yourself in a sticky situation, get out of there as quickly as you can. Find a quiet place to retreat to and find your center of serenity.

6. Take a moment to meditate. Your DNA may change dramatically and instantly if you can connect with your inner self.

These small behavioral changes have a big impact on your body's internal operations quickly. Your cells are appreciative on the inside, even though it might not be apparent on the outside.

Make your lifestyle valuable because it is essentially a direct communication between your body's genetic activity and you! This year, set a goal to not only fit into the slender blue jeans

that you've never seen before but also to pay
attention to the genes that make you, well, YOU.

Chapter 5:

Fit-Genes Customized Genetic Health and Wellbeing Assessment

Our approach to taking care of our bodies is getting more and more individualized as we strive for the best possible personal health. To the extent that a genetic specialist can now analyze your DNA and make dietary, exercise, and behavioral recommendations.
Allow me to introduce you to the exciting world of genetic profiling and nutrigenomics if, like me, you're interested in learning how to age well, eat healthily, and exercise responsibly.

What is genetic profiling precisely?

Genetic profiling is the study of an individual's genes (inherited from your mum and dad). The instructions for producing proteins, which are the building blocks of your body, are found in genes, which are little segments of DNA found throughout the genome.

These genes are in charge of giving you unique characteristics like eye color and height. Through gene research, we can also predict your susceptibility to particular traits and potential disorders.

What is Nutrigenomics exactly?

"This is where things start to get interesting." Nutrigenomics, to put it simply, is the study of the interactions between your genes and nutrients, or diets. Good lifestyle and eating choices help send 'healthy' signals to your genes, but poor choices can damage the DNA in your genes. Thus, you bring not only your hunger but also your DNA when we sit down to dinner. You can choose foods and lifestyle choices that lower your risk of obesity, diabetes, heart disease, cancer, and many other diseases once we know your genetic profile. What a freeing concept!

Genetic profiling can provide answers to a variety of issues, including:

- Do my genes make me more likely to acquire weight.
- Is coffee good for me?
- Can I benefit from fasting?
- Which kind of exercise is better for me: low- or high-intensity?
- Are the genes that make me more prone to inflammation?
- Do my genes have an impact on my mental health?
- Why can't I lose weight while following a low-fat or low-carb diet?
- How far along is my inherited ability to detoxify?
- To what degree can I tolerate stress?
- Is my likelihood of having higher LDL and lower HDL higher?

Knowing your personal nutrigenomic profile gives you the ability to make choices that lower your risk of disease and enhance your overall health and well-being. You can make up for genetic differences with the help of nutrigenomics.

Nutrigenomics is the "how"; genetics is the "what". It suggests evidence-based dietary, lifestyle, and exercise modifications to assist in modifying your genes' expression.

"Your genes do not determine your fate."

Even if your genes have remained the same throughout your life, you can alter the rate at which the enzymes they code for by adopting the right dietary and lifestyle choices. You hold the power.

Everybody has both genetic advantages and weaknesses; there are no "good" and "bad" genes. How they manifest in our lives is something we have to decide.

How are genetic tests performed?

Just a little swab from the inside of the cheek will do. It's an incredibly simple method. After testing your sample, I will provide you with a thorough health plan that is as distinct as your DNA along with a report.

Fit-Genes: Why Use It?

An increasing number of businesses are now providing this service due to the growing interest in nutrigenomics and genetic profiling. I selected 'Fit-Genes,' an Australian company, for a number of reasons.

First off, Fit-Genes only examines genes whose recommended actions are supported by a significant body of research.

Fit-Genes' interventions are not influenced by any supplements because the company has no affiliations with any of them.

Lastly, FitGenes provides a comprehensive and easy-to-use report that explores the importance of 62 distinct genes to human health.

FitGenes, in my opinion, is among the top companies that analyze DNA for health and wellness because of these criteria.

What the FitGenes report looks at: The genes that are analyzed include those that impact fat and cholesterol metabolism, cell defense, inflammation, vitamin D receptors, methylation, and homocysteine production (which are involved in mental well-being and energy production, including both common variants of the MTHFR genetic mutation), and cardiovascular health.

Chapter 6:

How to Clean Your Genes with the Soak and Scrub Method

Your genes are tainted. All of us are guilty of it. But a lot of individuals don't know that you can clean up your genetic makeup. You can influence how your body expresses its genes to promote optimal function. In short, you have the power to turn off genes that are detrimental to your health and turn on ones that are beneficial.

This explains how epigenetics works. Nutrigenomics and epigenetics will shape genetic studies in the future. Although they are scientific ideas, they can also seem otherworldly. This is due to the fact that implementing these concepts can actually change your genetic destiny.

By harnessing the power of nutrigenomics and epigenetics, you may help your genes express themselves in a way that works for you rather than against you.

Giving your genes what they need to express themselves best may allow you to rewrite the history of your health.

It's as simple as that! Your genes may be twisted, yet you might still be in good health.

How would one approach this? Dr. Ben Lynch's groundbreaking and internationally acclaimed book, Unclean Genes, walks you through the process of cleaning up your genetic mess. The soak-and-scrub approach is what is meant by this.

Have you started the book but not yet finished reading it? Maybe you read Dirty Genes before and need a recap of the Soak and Scrub?

This is all the information you need to start clearing your genetic history.

Dirty Genes Are Originated

Everybody has genetic SNPs (single nucleotide polymorphisms), also referred to as variances or mutations. Dr. Ben Lynch sometimes refers to these genes as "born dirty Genes."

You may be more prone to various health issues due to particular genes. For instance, a mutation in the MTHFR gene increases the likelihood of excessive homocysteine levels and folate deficiency, two conditions that are risk factors for cardiovascular disease. However, you can significantly reduce these risks by maintaining a clean MTHFR gene.

Your distinct genetic makeup is inherited from your parents. You inherit one set of chromosomes from your mother and one from your father. The precise chromosomes inherited from each parent influence your genetic makeup. When you inherit your parents' DNA, there are a lot of possible combinations.

Assume that your father carries two copies of the MTHFR C677T homozygous mutation. There are only two to select from, so he'll give you one for sure. Your mother is homozygous (has one copy) for MTHFR A1298C but lacks MTHFR C677T. She also has a non-variant choice, so she might or might not forward this to you.

One useful method for figuring out whether your genes were "dirty" or varied from birth is genetic testing. Making sense of your DNA test findings can be aided by using a thorough genetic analysis, like the StrateGene® DNA Report.

Let's say you find out you have two copies of the MTHFR C677T genetic variant. This would enable
You have homozygous MTHFR C677T. You are considered compound heterozygous for MTHFR if you have one copy of MTHFR and one copy of MTHFR A1298C. These two situations represent instances of "dirty MTHFR" genes that were contaminated from birth.

Remember that everyone possesses some genetic variation before you lose your mind. If we didn't, we would all be identical duplicates of one another! You can also take particular steps to clean your body of a born-dirty gene, such as a dirty MTHFR gene.

Methylation and MTHFR

Your lifestyle and experiences influence how your genes manifest themselves, in addition to genetic variants. A pure gene may get tainted during your lifetime. Poor nutrition, poor exercise routines, poor breathing patterns, ambient contaminants, and stress can all pollute a single gene. A born clean gene that becomes dirty owing to poor lifestyle choices can function similarly to a born dirty gene!

The StrataGene® DNA Report reveals that certain lifestyle variables, such as folic acid, can contaminate the MTHFR gene. Folic acid is an inadequate alternative for vitamin B9 (folate), which is required for methylation activities. A dirty MTHFR gene, whether it was unclean at birth or dirty, can inhibit the methylation cycle.

The biological process of methylation is simply defined as the activation of activities in your body by the transfer of carbon and hydrogen atoms to other substances.
Your methylation cycle must be functioning in order to express DNA. And, for methylation to occur, your MTHFR gene must be activated in order to produce MTHFR enzymes!

Methylation is a key step in the process of cleaning up your genes. When your genes act up or cause symptoms, it usually indicates that your methylation process isn't working properly. This is typically due to B12 and folate deficits produced by a defective MTHFR gene. Given that over half of the population is thought to have an MTHFR gene mutation, it's worthwhile to get tested to determine if you're one of them! (4) To support appropriate methylation processes in your body, you can take particular steps to clean your MTHFR genes, such as supplementing with methylated folate and methyl B12.

Do You Need To Clean Your Genes?

The majority of people will benefit from frequent gene cleaning. Modern life exposes us to more chemicals and toxins than our bodies have ever encountered. This can make our 'born clean DNA' unclean.

The vast majority of people have more than one genetic variant. You could have several distinct genes that are either born unclean or act dirty. Furthermore, your genes do not live in a vacuum. How one individual works has a wide-ranging impact. When one or more of them become contaminated, it can result in a wide range of difficulties, from minor symptoms to chronic diseases and everything in between.

While you can't change your genetic code, you can impact how your genes work by cleaning them regularly.

"Your genes are not your destiny," says Dr. Ben Lynch. This is because cleaning your DNA on a regular basis promotes good health. By giving targeted support, you can achieve the same results as if your MTHFR or other filthy genes were born clean.

Here's some more good news: cleansing one gene has a positive impact on other genes. While our bodies contain over 30,000 genes, Dr. Ben Lynch discovered that only a small number of them had a substantial impact on our health. These genetic variations are collectively referred to as the "Super Seven Genes."

Your 7 Super Genes

Although your body has hundreds of genes, these seven have the most significant impact on your health. If any of your Super Seven Genes is dirty, whether they were born unclean or are merely acting dirty, the rest of your genes will suffer.

Your Super Seven Genes are listed below:

1. MTHFR — Promotes methylation, which is required for over 200 of your body's essential functions, including genetic expression.

2. DAO — Alters your body's sensitivity to histamine from food and bacteria, increasing your susceptibility to allergy symptoms and food intolerance.

3. MAOA — Affects the interactions between dopamine, norepinephrine, and serotonin, influencing your mood, energy, sleep, and sugar cravings.

4. COMT - Controls the metabolism of important neurotransmitters that affect your mood, estrogen, and energy levels, as well as your ability to relax, sleep, and concentrate.

5. GST/GPX – Helps the body detoxify and cleanse itself of harmful toxins.

6. NOS3 — affects circulation and cardiovascular health.

7. PEMT - Affects your cell walls, brain, and liver, resulting in a variety of health issues such as pregnancy complications, fatty liver, digestive issues, and others.

Each of these genes has a unique set of functions and roles. Many of them create enzymes that power or support important biochemical and physiological processes. They have various consequences on your health. However, if they are dirty, they might have a negative impact on your quality of life.

Certain filthy genes are tough to clean. Not any of the seven. They are easily corrected with dietary and lifestyle changes. The tricky part is deciding which of your Super Seven Genes are filthy and need help. These genes have slightly different optimization needs. Dr. Ben Lynch developed a test to help you determine which of your Super Seven Genes is acting up. The entire assessment can be read in his book, Dirty Genes. You can also get a shorter online version here.

How Do Genes Accumulate Dirt?

Your DNA can be polluted in a number of ways. It is possible to be born with "dirty" variants, such as the MTHFR cases listed above.
You can have clean genes that become dirty as a result of environmental or lifestyle exposures like heavy metals, secondhand smoke, workplace chemical exposure, major stress or trauma, and so on.
The good news is that your DNA isn't fixed. You can also clean them if they've become dirty. Regardless of the type of genetic diversity you have, the basic method of cleansing your DNA remains applicable. However, it must be adjusted to your particular symptoms and needs.

You are unlike anyone else in any aspect of health. You should use these unique notions in your case.

Discover how to clean your DNA in six simple steps.

Clean your genes in 6 easy steps.

Your genetics are unique. So, how can software work for so many people when our DNA is so diverse?

The Soak and Scrub technique, detailed by Dr. Ben Lynch in Dirty Genes, is meant to cleanse your genetic health over the course of two weeks. To function properly, all genes must follow the same healthy behaviors.

Scrub and soak.

Soak and Scrub is a fundamental concept. It's an opportunity to reconnect with your body and press the reset button. By addressing the various aspects of your lifestyle, you lay the foundations for your best health by giving your genes the support they need to function without interruption.

A Soak and Scrub is not meant to be a rigorous diet or way of life. It's a fresh start. It is time to cleanse and refuel. It's time to clear out the cobwebs and get rid of brain fog, among other things.

It will not occur by itself. You need to be strategic in five crucial areas:

- Food\sSupplements\sDetoxification
- Stress Reduction through Sleep

These are the core components required for good health, regardless of inherited issues. When we neglect one or more of these areas in our hectic and busy modern world, we become fatigued, ill, nervous, annoyed, and less than ideal.

Here's an overview of how to use the Soak and Scrub to cleanse your genes:

1. Remove any obstructions

First and foremost, before making any decision, consider, "Will this make my genes work harder?"

Before you start cleansing your genes, eliminate any obstructions that will make the process more difficult. Examine your lifestyle from a strategic perspective. The Soak and Scrub approach is designed to get your clean DNA program started. It is intended to last two weeks, but you may prolong or adapt it to meet your specific needs.

You go on vacation to unwind and refresh. Consider a Soak and Scrub as the same thing for your DNA. Of course, you can't simply turn your genes off to restart them. However, aggravating factors can be removed.

A Soak and Scrub include foods, supplements, and lifestyle choices that support your detox organs (liver, kidneys, and lungs). However, before we get into each individual topic, consider the following:

- Is there anything I can remove from my calendar for the next two weeks?
- Can you go on a literal work vacation?
- Can you refuse certain commitments?
- Can you limit your smartphone and device usage to allow your brain more time to recharge?

- Is there anything I know I need more of?
- Do you drink enough water each day?
- Do you participate in regular physical activity?

2. Food Nutrigenomics.

Food Nutrigenomics is the study of how your genes react to diet and nutrition. You do not have to follow a rigorous diet. However, you must ensure that your body gets the nourishment it needs to restore its methylation processes and DNA expression. That is a crucial part of the Soak and Scrub regimen.

Gut health and the microbiome have a significant impact on gene expression. They establish the foundation for how your cells, tissues, and organs perform. Probiotics represent only one component of intestinal health. Everything you consume, digest, and absorb is included.

The biggest way that eating influences your Soak and Scrub is to pay attention to how it makes you feel. When you think about it, many of the foods you eat for convenience, pleasure, or enjoyment may actually be causing digestive problems that are harmful to your health.

The specific foods for you may vary, but common dietary triggers include:

- Gluten\sDairy
- Fried foods
- Prepared foods.
- Sugar\sSoy
- Wine, cheese, chocolate, and cured meats are all high in histamines.

This does not mean you must avoid trigger foods eternally. However, during a Soak and Scrub, you want to reduce any noise. You want to remove anything that is interfering with your desired gene expression.

Do you plan your meals? Even if you aren't, creating a meal plan for your Soak and Scrub can help you unwind when it's time to eat.

Your finances can influence your eating habits. However, eating well doesn't have to be excessively expensive. Take your grocery budget and purchase the finest quality foods you can locate. Make use of your local farmers market. Buy staples in bulk. Make modest modifications, such as serving roasted vegetables as a side dish instead of white rice.

Additional food ideas for your Soak and Scrub:

- Begin with a whole-food diet high in protein and healthy fats.
- Eliminate cow's milk dairy, gluten, excess carbs, and white sugar from your diet.
- When possible, select organic foods.
- Avoid snacks and late-night meals until you're 80% satisfied.
- Only eat when you are hungry. Do not nibble just because you have a habit, are fatigued, or are concerned. Ask yourself how you feel and what your body needs.
- Fast for 12 to 16 hours each day. This is simple to accomplish if you eat a later dinner and breakfast.
- Eat gently and thoroughly. Chewing more makes digestion easier.

- Drink your beverages in between meals, not during them.
- Adjust your diet to include or exclude foods that are suitable for your genetic composition.

3. Additions.

It is ideal to get all of your nutrients from meals. But in today's world, that isn't always possible. This is feasible due of:

Critical minerals have been removed from soils.

Harvesting crops before they reach their peak and exporting them throughout the world has become common practice, as opposed to consuming foods that are at their peak and in season. Cooking procedures might deplete some nutrients.

Shelf life can alter nutrient levels.

Individual digestive and physiological conditions influence absorption rates.

However, just because supplements can be healthy does not imply you should take them in large quantities. What works well for you may not be successful for another. More of a good thing is not always preferable.

When it comes to vitamins, there are several factors to consider.

As previously mentioned, folate is essential for methylation. However, folate is not the same as folic acid. There are several forms of folate. Nutrients may be bioavailable or "active" in general.

Alternatively, they may require your body to transform them into forms that can be used in a variety of ways. This can make your genes work harder, which is not ideal for a Soak and Scrub. The type of supplement greatly influences how well it is absorbed by your body. Always choose supplements that are the most bioavailable, or active chemical forms.

Supplements come in various forms, including capsules, lozenges, liquids, liposomes, powders, chewables, and tinctures. Use the form that best meets your needs. Liposomal formulations are frequently the easiest to absorb, whereas pills are the most difficult.

Always follow your doctor's advice regarding dosage. You can also use the pulse technique to calculate how much you need and when to increase, decrease, or discontinue the dose completely. This expands on the idea of listening to your body. You can take the supplement whenever you feel your body needs extra support. However, on a good day, your body may not need it. The pulse strategy does not work for every supplement, but it does for the majority of them.

Prenatal vitamins, multivitamins, electrolytes, probiotics, glutathione, and methyl folate are some of the most commonly used supplements to support all dirty genes. Dr. Ben Lynch's supplement recommendations for all Super Seven genes are listed below. These are starting points to help you achieve optimum genetic well-being.

4. Detoxification

Detoxification is not a gimmick. People who want to offer you unproven things may misuse the term, but the process is a biological fact. You have organs that assist with the detoxification process. These include the liver, kidneys, bladder, intestines, lungs, and even the skin.

Your immune system, cardiovascular system, and other systems are dependent on your body's ability to clear waste. Every day, you are exposed to toxins through the air you breathe, the food you eat, and the surroundings you live in. This cannot be avoided. Our bodies were not designed to endure this chemical burden, which has a harmful influence on our DNA. To fully support your body, maximize your detox organs and detoxification pathways.

When your genes are faulty and your methylation is weak, your body's detoxification ability suffers.

By using some basic strategies during your Soak and Scrub, you can reduce the burden that your body has to detox from.

Instead of plastic or nonstick cookware, use stainless steel, glass, ceramic, or cast iron.
Remove any air fresheners, synthetic scents, or fragrances from your home.
Avoid using pesticides, insecticides, or herbicides. When possible, select organic foods.
Take adequate care of mold, mildew, damp areas in your home, and other environmental contaminants.
Sweating a much. Exercise, baths, saunas, and hot showers can all help with detoxification.

5. Sleep

Rest is a crucial aspect of overall wellness. This is because the majority of your body's healing occurs when you sleep! If you are having trouble sleeping or simply do not appreciate it sufficiently as a result of the hustling culture, it is time to rethink your priorities. Sleep is critical for preserving healthy genes. When you sleep, your body enters a state of rest and restoration, preparing it for the next day.

Here are some Soak and Scrub recommendations to improve your sleep hygiene:

- To maintain a consistent sleep/wake cycle, go to bed at the same time every day, no later than 10:30 p.m.
- To maintain a healthy circadian rhythm, which is required for sufficient hormone synthesis and balance, you must get enough sleep (7 to 8 hours) on a consistent schedule.
- To achieve perfect darkness, turn off or block all artificial lights at night and in your bedroom. A good sleep mask could also assist with this.
- By 2 p.m., you should have ceased drinking coffee (or quit drinking it completely).
- Turn off all the displays. 1–2 hours before bedtime.

- Before going to bed, practice deep breathing, meditation, or other soothing activities.

If you're having difficulties sleeping and are continually tired, consult your doctor or a naturopath. You could have sleep apnea or other disorders that are interfering with your body's ability to get deep.

Restorative sleep. Consider consulting with your healthcare professional about further sleep aids.

6. Anxiety

The world is a challenging environment! There is no getting around that. However, you can take steps to lower your risks.

Stress, in any form, can have a significant negative impact on your health by weakening your immune system, making weight loss difficult, and causing inflammation.

Stress can result from a multitude of factors. Many people are stressed on several fronts. Food can worsen stress, especially if you are sensitive to or intolerant to histamines. Environmental variables can cause stress if you are overstimulated all the time. Workplace and personal relationships may both be difficult.

You may not be able to address all stressors during your two-week Soak and Scrub, but identifying them is the first step toward protecting your health.

If you don't know where to start, here are some tips for minimizing stress during your Soak and Scrub:

- Say "no" more often.
- Get outside every day to breathe fresh air and relax.
- Every day, spend at least five minutes meditating, practicing yoga, or stretching.
- Deep breathing should be practiced. Breathe softly and steadily through your nose, not your mouth.
- Get the right amount of exercise for your body—not too much or too little. Excessive exercise, particularly when

weary or unwell, can be a major source of stress.

Chapter 7

Heart Problems: What Exactly is Heart Disease (Cardiovascular)?

The heart, like any other muscle in the body, requires a sufficient blood supply to provide oxygen to the muscle, allowing it to contract and pump blood throughout the body. The heart not only pumps blood throughout the body, but it also pumps blood into itself via the coronary arteries. These arteries come from the base of the aorta (the main blood vessel that delivers oxygenated blood from the heart) and branch out along its surface.

When one or more coronary arteries narrow, adequate blood flow to the heart becomes difficult, particularly during exercise. This can cause the heart muscle, like any other muscle in the body, to ache. If the arteries continue to thin, exercise may be insufficient to stress the heart and induce symptoms. Angina is characterized by chest pain or pressure, as well as shortness of breath, which frequently radiates to the shoulders, arms, and/or neck.

If one of the coronary arteries gets completely clogged, usually as a result of a plaque rupture that causes a blood clot to form, blood flow to a section of the heart may be interrupted. This causes the demise of a portion of the heart muscle. This results in a heart attack, commonly known as a myocardial infarction (**myo=muscle + cardia=heart + infarction=tissue death**).

For the purposes of this article, cardiovascular disease is defined as a spectrum of atherosclerosis or arterial hardening ranging from a modest blockage with no symptoms to a complete obstruction with myocardial infarction. Other topics, such as myocarditis, heart valve problems, and congenital heart defects, should be avoided.

Symptoms of cardiovascular (heart) disease

1. Angina, often known as heart pain, is characterized by a crushing pressure or heaviness in the middle of the chest, which radiates to the arm (typically the left) or jaw. You may experience shortness of breath, sweating, and nausea.

2. Symptoms are typically started by activity and improve with rest.

3. Some people may have indigestion and nausea, but others may feel pain in their upper belly, shoulders, or back.

4. Unstable angina is defined as feelings that occur at rest, wake the patient, and do not respond quickly to nitroglycerin or rest.

Chapter 8:

Symptoms and causes of heart problems

"Heart disease" refers to any disorder that negatively affects the cardiovascular system. There are several types, some of which are avoidable.

According to the Centers for Disease Control and Prevention (CDC), heart disease is the leading cause of mortality in the United States. Heart disease kills around one in every four people in the United States and affects all genders, races, and ethnicities.

This article explains the various forms, causes, and symptoms of heart disease. This page also addresses risk factors and treatment alternatives. Symptoms The symptoms of heart disease differ according to the type. Furthermore, certain heart problems produce no symptoms at all.

However, the following indicators may indicate a heart problem:

angina or chest pain, trouble breathing, tiredness, lightheadedness, edema, or swelling caused by fluid retention
Cyanosis, or a blue tinge to the skin, and difficulties exercising are indicators of a congenital heart defect in children.

Here are some indications and symptoms of a heart attack:
Symptoms may include chest discomfort, shortness of breath, palpitations in the heart, stomach ache, nausea, arm, jaw, back, or leg pain from sweating, a sense of suffocation, and fatigue from swelling ankles.
An irregular heartbeat
A heart attack can cause cardiac arrest, which is when the heart stops beating and the body becomes unable to function. If a person

experiences any of the signs of a heart attack, they should seek emergency medical attention.

Reasons and potential threats of heart disease.

The following conditions can cause cardiac disease:

Possible causes of cardiac problems include injury, blood artery issues, decreased oxygen and nutrition intake, and disruptions in heart rhythm.

In some cases, the disorder may be genetically determined. However, a variety of lifestyle variables and medical conditions may raise the risk. These include the following:

- Hypertension; high blood pressure.
- Smoking raises cholesterol.
- Excessive alcohol consumption is associated with overweight and obesity. Diabetes, family history of cardiovascular disease.

- Nutrition, age, and a history of preeclampsia during pregnancy are all factors to consider.
- Lower levels of activity
- Sleep apnea
- High amounts of tension and anxiety.
- Leaking heart valves

According to the World Health Organization (WHO), Trusted Source poverty and stress are two of the major factors contributing to an increase in heart and cardiovascular disease globally.

Treatments

Modifying one's lifestyle, taking medication, and having surgery are all common treatment options for heart disease; however, the specific treatments accessible to a patient will vary based on the type of cardiac condition that they have.

In the following sections, we will go over several of these alternatives in greater detail.

Medications

A vast range of medications.

Heart problems can be managed with the help of a trusted source. The primary choices are as follows:

Anticoagulants are medications that can prevent blood clots; they are also known as blood thinners. They include the direct oral anticoagulants dabigatran, rivaroxaban, and

Apixaban and warfarin (brand name Coumadin) are both blood thinners.

Antiplatelet therapy, such as aspirin and other similar drugs, can help avoid blood clots.

Angiotensin-converting enzyme inhibitors are a class of medications that can be used to treat both heart failure and excessive blood pressure. These drugs act by widening the blood vessels. One such example is the medication lisinopril.

Another way to lower blood pressure is to use angiotensin II receptor blockers. One example is the medication losartan.

Angiotensin receptor neprilysin inhibitors are drugs that have the ability to help the heart unload and disrupt the molecular mechanisms that cause weakening.

Metoprolol and other medications in this class, known as beta-blockers, can reduce the heart rate and lower blood pressure. They are also useful in treating arrhythmias and angina.

Calcium channel blockers are a type of drug that can relax blood vessels and reduce the force with which the heart pumps blood, so decreasing blood pressure and lowers the risk of arrhythmias. Diltiazem is one such medicine (Cardizem).

Statins, such as atorvastatin (Lipitor), and other types of medications can help reduce the amount of low-density lipoprotein cholesterol in the body.

The force with which the heart pumps blood around the body can be considerably increased by employing preparations such as digoxin (Lanoxin). They are also effective in treating cardiac failure and arrhythmias.

Diuretics are medications that lower blood pressure, reduce the burden on the heart, and remove excess water from the body. Diuretics are commonly known as "water pills." Furosemide (Lasix) is an example.

Vasodilators are a family of medications used to treat excessive blood pressure. They accomplish this by lowering blood vessel stress. One example is nitroglycerin, often known as Nitrostat. These medications may also help relieve chest pain. Read on for more information on vasodilation.

Chapter 9:

Role of Nutrition in Gene Optimization

Nutrition has a significant impact on our entire health, influencing not only our energy levels and weight but also the fundamental foundation of our being - our genes. When it comes to filthy genes, the role of nutrition in gene optimization becomes even more important. In this exploration, we'll look at essential foods that can positively influence gene expression, and we'll discover how modest dietary decisions can have a big impact on our health.

The Foundation

Let us start with the basics. A gene-friendly diet is not about limitation; it's about feeding. It is about giving our bodies the necessary building ingredients to promote effective gene expression. At its heart, this entails eating a well-balanced mix of macronutrients (proteins, fats, and carbohydrates) as well as a diverse range of micronutrients.

Proteins: The Architects of Gene Health

Proteins are our bodies' workhorses, engaging in a wide range of cellular functions. Certain amino acids stand out during gene optimization. Methionine and cysteine, for example, are sulfur-containing amino acids that are essential for DNA methylation, which affects gene activity. Foods high in these amino acids, such as poultry, fish, eggs, and legumes, are critical components of a gene-friendly diet.

Healthy Fats: Fueling the Genetic Machinery

Not all fats are created equal, and choosing the proper fats can help optimize gene function. Omega-3 fatty acids, which are plentiful in fatty fish such as salmon, flaxseeds, and walnuts, help to reduce inflammation and promote healthy gene expression. These lipids work as lubricants for the genetic machinery, keeping it running smoothly.

Complex Carbohydrates: Maintaining Genetic Harmony

carbs frequently receive a poor rap, although complex carbs are an essential source of energy for our bodies. Whole grains, fruits, and vegetables give a consistent supply of glucose, which is our cells' primary energy source. This prolonged energy promotes a balanced environment for gene expression, avoiding the unpredictable spikes and crashes associated with refined carbohydrates.

Micronutrients: Small But Mighty

While macronutrients provide the groundwork, micronutrients are the unsung heroes, little in number but powerful in impact. These vitamins and minerals function as cofactors and coenzymes, aiding a variety of metabolic activities required for gene optimization.

Vitamin D: The Sunshine Vitamin for Genes.

Consider vitamin D to be the sunshine your genes seek. It controls the expression of several genes, including those involved in immunological function and cell proliferation. Exposure to sunlight and vitamin D-rich meals such as fatty fish and fortified dairy products guarantees that your genes benefit from this crucial mineral.

Vitamin B: The B's and C's of Genetic Support

The B-vitamin family, which includes B6, B12, and folate, is essential for methylation processes, which constitute an important element of gene control. Leafy greens, lentils, and lean meats are high in B vitamins. Furthermore, vitamin C is a powerful antioxidant, protecting your genes from oxidative damage and promoting general genetic integrity.

Minerals Provide Crystalline Support for Genomic Stability.

Minerals like zinc and magnesium serve as crystalline pillars, ensuring the stability of your genetic system. Zinc, found in seeds, nuts, and red meat, helps with DNA repair, whereas magnesium, found in leafy greens and whole grains, contributes to the overall structural integrity of your genes.

Plant Nutrients: Nature's Genetic Elixirs

Nature offers us a wealth of phytonutrients, plant components that not only give fruits and vegetables their brilliant colors but also provide several health advantages.

Polyphenols: Colorful Guardians of Genetic Integrity

Polyphenols present in berries, tea, and dark chocolate protect genomic integrity. They influence gene expression, providing antioxidant and anti-inflammatory benefits that spread across your genetic profile.

Sulforaphane, Broccoli's Genetic Superhero
Sulforaphane, a chemical found in broccoli and other cruciferous vegetables, promotes the development of phase II enzymes, which aid in the detoxification of toxic compounds. This superhero vitamin shows how dietary choices can favorably influence gene expression.

Nutrition for Gene Optimization: Revealing the Secrets to a Healthier You.

Key Nutrients For Dirty Genes

Genes, like silent conductors, react to the symphony of nutrients we supply through our food. Understanding these critical actors enables targeted gene optimization.

1. Omega-3 Fatty Acids: Nourish the Genetic Orchestra

Omega-3 fatty acids, which are rich in fatty fish, flaxseeds, and walnuts, play key roles in the genetic symphony. They have anti-inflammatory properties, which attenuate the discordant tones that may result from gene malfunction. According to research, they can help reduce the risk of a variety of ailments, including cardiovascular disease and mood disorders.

2. Antioxidants: Protectors against Genetic Stress

Our genes are continually under stress from external influences. Antioxidants, found in colorful fruits and vegetables, serve as attentive guardians. They neutralize free radicals, keeping them from causing havoc with our genetic code. Incorporating a variety of plant-based diets provides a varied range of antioxidants to strengthen our genetic defenses.

3. Methyl Donors for Fine-Tuning Gene Expression

Methyl donors, like as folate, B vitamins, and choline, act as precise artisans in gene expression. They bind methyl groups to genes, regulating their activity. Ensuring a proper supply of essential nutrients is analogous to applying the subtle brushstrokes that transform a canvas - in this case, our genetic landscape.

4. Polyphenols: Nature's Elixir of Gene Harmony

Polyphenols, which can be found in tea, red wine, dark chocolate, and a range of fruits and vegetables, help to balance our DNA. Their varied set of chemicals has protective properties, increasing genetic stability and resilience. The interaction of polyphenols with our genes emphasizes the need to eat a diverse, plant-based diet.

Practical Strategies for A Gene-Friendly Diet

With an understanding of critical nutrients, creating a gene-friendly diet becomes a tangible path to greater health. Practical solutions provide the framework for effectively incorporating these nutrients into our daily lives.

1. Diversify Your Plate: A Palette of Nutritious Foods

The foundation of a gene-friendly diet is diversity. Strive for a rainbow of hues on your plate, representing a diverse array of nutrients. To ensure nutrient balance, eat a variety of fruits, vegetables, whole grains, and lean proteins.

2. Mindful Meal Planning: Balancing Macronutrients to Promote Gene Harmony

When macronutrients - proteins, lipids, and carbs - are balanced, meal planning becomes an art form. Each macronutrient adds its own notes to the genetic symphony. Choose lean proteins, healthy fats, and complex carbohydrates to produce a symphony that promotes proper gene expression.

3. Seasonal and Local: Natural Rhythms in Your Diet

Embrace the seasonal wealth that nature delivers. Seasonal and regionally obtained foods not only have high nutritional value, but they also follow the natural rhythms of our environment. By matching our diets to the changing seasons, we improve our genetic adaptation and resilience.

4. Cooking Methods Matter: Maintaining Nutrient Integrity

The way we prepare food affects its nutritious content. Choose cooking methods that maintain the integrity of vital nutrients. Steaming, sautéing, and baking are gentle processes that preserve the nutritious value of foods, ensuring that our genes reap the full range of benefits.

Meal Plans and Recipes

Going on a gene-friendly diet does not entail giving up the thrill of tasty food. Let's look at a day's worth of meal ideas and recipes that highlight the confluence of taste and genetic well-being.

1. Breakfast: Omega-3-Boosting Smoothies

Ingredients: - 1 cup mixed berries (blueberries and strawberries) - 1 tablespoon ground flaxseeds.

- One-half banana
- One cup of almond milk.
- A handful of spinach (optional for an added nutritional boost).

Instructions:

- Blend all the ingredients until smooth.
- Pour into a glass and enjoy the omega-3 benefits.

2. Lunch: Mediterranean Quinoa Salad.

Ingredients: - 1 cup cooked quinoa - Cherry tomatoes, cucumber, and diced red bell pepper
- Kalamata olives and feta cheese are optional.
- Fresh lemon vinaigrette (olive oil, lemon juice, garlic, oregano).

Instructions:
- Combine all items in a bowl.
- Drizzle with lemon vinaigrette for a Mediterranean-style genetic feast.

3. Dinner: Baked Salmon and Herbed Sweet Potatoes
Ingredients include salmon fillets, sweet potatoes (sliced), olive oil, garlic, rosemary, and thyme. - Lemon wedges to serve.

Instructions:
- Season fish with herbs and bake until flaky.

- Roast sweet potato slices with olive oil and garlic.
- Serve with a squeeze of lemon for a nutritious meal.

Common Misconceptions About Nutrition and Genes

Dispelling common myths is critical when navigating the complex world of nutrition and genetics. Let us unravel the truths that are frequently veiled by misinformation.

1. Misconception: "Genetics Determines Everything"

- Truth: Although genetics play an important role, lifestyle factors such as food can have a substantial impact on gene expression. Our choices have the ability to influence genetic outcomes.

2. Misconception: "One Size Fits All" Nutrition

- Truth: Each person's genetic makeup is unique. A personalized approach to nutrition takes into account genetic variations, ensuring that nutritional recommendations are appropriate for each individual.

3. Misconception: "Nutrition Has No Impact on Gene Expression"

- Nutrition functions as a dynamic switchboard, regulating the activity of our genes. Nutrient-dense diets give the signals that direct our genes toward peak performance.

4. Misconception: "Genetic Predisposition Is Destiny"

- Truth: While genetics influence predispositions, lifestyle decisions can change the course. A gene-friendly diet and healthy practices can reduce genetic risks while increasing resilience.

In the symphony of nutrition and gene optimization, every decision we make contributes to the great composition of our well-being. We set out on a mission to become a healthier, gene-optimized self, armed with knowledge, practical tactics, and delicious meals. Let the gastronomic alchemy begin as we enjoy the harmony of nutrients that dance in sync with our genetic orchestra.